Scrolls in the Wilderness

Thanks for the Donation! *Luke Rideout*

Scrolls in the Wilderness

*A Guide to Healing and Spiritual Warfare
from the Essenes*

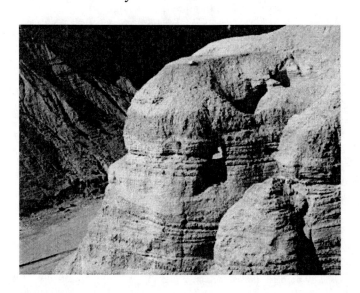

KATHLEEN ARAI
AND
LUKE RIDEOUT

WIPF & STOCK · Eugene, Oregon

SCROLLS IN THE WILDERNESS
A Guide to Healing and Spiritual Warfare from the Essenes

Wipf and Stock Publishers
199 W. 8th Ave., Suite 3
Eugene, OR 97401

www.wipfandstock.com

ISBN 13: 978-1-60608-059-7

Scripture quotations taken from the New American Standard Bible®, Copyright © 1960, 1962, 1963, 1968, 1971, 1972, 1973, 1975, 1977, 1995 by The Lockman Foundation Used by permission. (www.Lockman.org).

Photograph from inside Qumran Cave 11 taken by John Sharpe. All other photographs are the property of Geoffrey Arai.

Manufactured in the U.S.A.

Dedicated to

Victor
A man who leads by example and love.
We love and admire you so much.

Glenn
For your kindness and dedication to family.
You and Mila are a blessing.

Benjamin
For your caring and humor. You have your priorities in order.
Both you and Corrie are not only family but also friends.

Geoffrey
For being the amazing fluffy. Sharing life experiences with
you has been an incredible pleasure. You bless and brighten
everywhere you go.

Kenley
The mad scientist, sharpfox, and wise young man.
For being loving and brilliant all at once!

With Special Thanks to

John Wipf
For his long-time valued friendship

Susan Carlson Wood
For incredible editing skills that helped us finally
make this book happen

John Sharpe
For being a good friend and sharing this journey with us

Christine Hughes
For her writing assistance

Contents

Photographs

Preface

THE PURPOSE of this book is to help the reader embrace the concept of healing as something created and ordained by God, not a recent concept or new discovery of the late twentieth century. We will review several manuscripts from the Dead Sea Scrolls that include material comparable to modern popular teachings of "spiritual warfare." As you read this book, you will begin to see a connection between the two. Thus, we will pull together the original intent of these documents and look at their implications for a person's life and for the world today.

Demons are real and present. They were for virtually everyone in first-century Palestine. However, current replacement theology and Western-worldview Christianity has taken the "historical knowledge" of this realm that was passed down through the ancients, particularly in the Hebrew Judaic world, and revamped it to look like something totally foreign and almost unrecognizable to Jesus himself.[1]

So we must look at information regarding spiritual warfare in the Second Temple Period (second century BCE to first century CE) in its context. Doing so will give better insight into the truth of genuine inner healing, and it will protect us from the idolatry of changing God into our image as opposed to letting him mold us into his.

---

1. References in this book to the Brit Hadasha/New Testament, Jesus, and Christian history are part of the authors' academic examination.

This book also gives a narrative—stories—to give the reader a sense of culture and environment. After all, this is what the ancients did best; they told stories. These stories have been created in partnership with Dead Sea Scroll references, with a focus on the Essenes. The Essenes were a significant community in the Judean wilderness during the Second Temple Period. Their members were intentionally set apart, not polluted or bombarded with the influence of multiple cultural beliefs systems. Thus, they give us a gift: tools and references for a life with protection and freedom. It is this gift that we hope you will receive through this book.

One

Rivka's Story

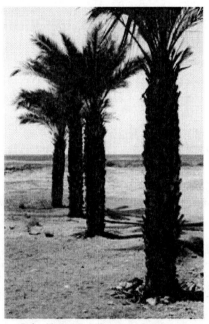

Palm Trees Near Qumran Community
at the Dead Sea

FLEEING FROM HOME

R IVKA PEERED around the corner before turning down each narrow street on her way to buy bread and vegetables. Like so many mornings, Roman soldiers appeared on the streets of Jerusalem and might accost you, insult you—or worse. More and more streamed into the city to put down the revolt against the Roman Empire. Rivka and her husband, Yosef, a Levite who assisted the priests in the Temple, sympathized with the revolt. But they also wondered if this was really the way that freedom would come. Shouldn't they be praying more for the coming of the Messiah? How could they defeat the Romans without the Messiah? But how could the Messiah come when the Temple was desecrated with Roman standards?

The same questions swirled through Rivka's mind as she hurried through the narrower alleys to the market street. She prayed that Yosef would be able to find a route to the Temple free from soldiers. How frustrated he felt when he was called to serve but then couldn't get to the Temple for fear of a beating from one of them in a bad mood.

That evening Rivka learned that Yosef had not tried to make it to the Temple that day. He had other errands. He also wanted to make sure that the journals they kept were finished and safely buried. Shortly after they were married Yosef began teaching Rivka to read and write so she could help in writing his journals. What a pleasure that had been for them to do together! But tonight Rivka felt a foreboding as he insisted they bury the scroll they had been working on recently.

When they finished, Yosef wrapped his cloak around Rivka. His eyes and ears were keen this night; he knew they had to escape; he had to save his family. This would be the night. Rivka held newborn Reuven to her breast as he held his daughter Elisheva's three-year-old hand. He loved holding her tiny hand, and as he did he memorized the feel of the shape, and promise of it.

Yosef could hear the onslaught of horses and Roman chariots up and down the streets of Jerusalem. His small family carried what they could as they left their humble home. Yosef remembered their last conversation before abandoning their home:

"Yosef, . . . why must we leave now? Where are we to go? How are we to survive?" Rivka's voice shook as she spoke. She had never been beyond the city and was frightened of what lay beyond what she knew.

"Rivka, don't you know that the Romans are destroying our city?" Yosef's tone was cool and calm as he tried to reason with his wife.

"They can't want us *all* dead . . . what purpose is that? Why aren't we at the Temple with everyone and praying to God and asking him for our salvation?" she scolded.

Yosef abruptly turned on her with anger in his voice, "Rivka, the Temple is not safe, the Romans are determined to destroy our Temple by burning it to the ground! Do you want our children burned alive? They won't care who's in the Temple, as long as it's ashes." His face carried his fury. He could not believe his wife, the mother of his children, would be so reckless, and not understand his plea to leave their beloved city.

He understood what was happening. The Romans invaded his country and were not satisfied with simply conquering and occupying the territory, as they called it, but they were determined to destroy Jerusalem.

Rivka was stricken. She had never seen her husband so angry. She then understood that she must do as he said and leave Jerusalem.

The Roman army led by Titus viciously confiscated food from the mouths of the men, women, and children of the city. Those who didn't die of starvation were sold into slavery, and sent to lands beyond the sun.

Days before, Yosef discovered that his brother and wife had died an agonizing death, each starving. Their children were sold and sent to Rome, never to be seen or heard from again. This fate was not going to befall his family.

Yosef had waited for nightfall to make the escape. With raw determination, he now fixed his eyes on Rivka. With Yosef's silent communication, Rivka knew this was the time to escape. She clutched her son Reuven closer and followed her husband out of their modest home.

The tiny family huddled together and slowly walked out of their home and into the street. Yosef, watchful of the soldiers, led his family in the direction out of Jerusalem. He silently prayed and begged God to rescue his family and lead them to safety.

As they made their way through the street, Yosef watched the movements of the Roman soldiers. He had spent the previous weeks studying their movements and routines. He moved his family when he felt sure it was safe.

Rivka felt Reuven stir and let go of Yosef's hand to comfort her son. She could see his face scrunching to howl. She knew if she did not act quickly to quiet her son, they would be found out. Rivka lifted Reuven to her breast so he could suckle and not cry out into the night.

Yosef turned abruptly when he discovered his freed hand and saw her, in one motion, quiet their son. Admiration and love for this woman filled Yosef—this woman who could instinctively know what to do in a desperate situation.

Each step was agony. Thoughts raced through his terrified mind: *What if we are caught? What will happen to my family? God, please lead us to salvation.*

As they crept through the city, their movements went undetected. The one soldier Yosef did see was filling his belly with stolen bread and wine, and they slipped by unnoticed.

The city gates were coming closer with each step. The family hid behind the wall of a home. Elisheva whimpered as she again knelt down on the hard ground. She was tired and her empty stomach grumbled. Yosef tightened his grip on his daughter's hand when she made the sound. His grip hurt, but when she looked up to her father, he was watching a soldier near the gates. She followed her father's line of vision and saw the man grab a boy and fling him into the dirt. The soldier kicked and beat him. Elisheva's eyes opened wide witnessing this savage beating. She opened her mouth to scream, but Yosef covered his daughter's mouth and eyes. He leaned over her to shield and comfort her from the sight of a bloody boy who lay lifeless in the street.

Satisfied with his handiwork, the soldier kicked the boy again to ensure the killing was complete and marched off to, likely, tell his friends of his entertainment.

Rivka shook at the sight and it roused Reuven. She lowered her head and murmured sweet sounds in his ear. Contented, Reuven closed his sleepy eyes.

Yosef knew that at any moment the gate would open for the caravan of merchants and tradesmen who came to the city each month. He had planned for this night since the last full moon. He observed the last caravan and knew that his family could get lost in the mix of people entering and make their escape.

Now was their chance. If they missed this, Yosef knew in his bones that his family wouldn't survive another week, let alone a month. He shuddered at the thought of his beautiful children sold as slaves, and he couldn't bring himself to think about what could happen to his beloved Rivka before the Roman monsters took her life.

When he decided the only option for his family's survival was to escape, he developed the plan. For two nights before he sat down with his wife and reviewed the plan; she knew what to do. The moment had come, now was the time to move. He winked at his wife, and she readied herself and their son for quick movement.

The city gate opened and the first of the caravans moved inside the city walls—the oxen and asses with their bulging packs of merchandise and supplies for sale. Ordinarily everyone in the city enjoyed the arrival of the caravans, but now the city population was quickly dwindling. The only reason for this caravan was to keep the soldiers supplied and their bellies full.

Yosef managed to acquire the right dress so he and his family could blend into the crowd. As they made their move, they went unnoticed among the oxen and asses, their packs so huge that the family could easily hide among them. Every hoof kicked up earth. The merchants looked past the little family; the few that took notice didn't give away Yosef or his family, for they knew what Yosef needed to do. Those eyes looked upon Yosef and Rivka with pity and concern. Each of the merchants knew that if the soldiers caught Yosef the penalty would be gruesome.

The city gate waited only steps away now, and Yosef could smell freedom. Rivka followed closely behind her husband, clutching their son and minding the steps of their daughter. It wasn't unusual for a small family to be among the merchants, as the merchants many times traveled with their families.

As they made their way to the gate, a voice shouted to them, "You there! No one goes outside the gate without a guard. Get back to your caravan!" the soldier yelled above the animals to Yosef. Panic filled his veins, what to do now? He hadn't planned to be seen. He had hoped that they would go unnoticed and that the soldiers wouldn't see one little family in the midst of all the animals and merchants. He looked at his wife, who was stricken with fear. When he looked back to the soldier, he heard another voice.

"Leave him, he is going to the next town to get more supplies for your troops. There are more oxen that need to be led back, and he is a trusted servant who will do this for me," the voice belonged to a white-haired man with a beard as long as Yosef's arm. This burly man spoke with such authority that Nero himself would have taken notice. This bearded man looked over at Yosef, and with one motion he waved Yosef off to do what was being asked of him.

Yosef could not believe his ears. Their eyes connected, and Yosef understood that this man knew that Yosef and his family were escaping.

The soldier looked bewildered, but nodded approval, and waved them through the gate. This Roman then turned his attention to the packs on the oxen, and tried to pull one down to ravage the contents.

Once beyond the city gate, the tiny family ran as fast as they could into the night. Yosef knew the territory well, as he had explored it with his brother when they were children. He followed the bright star to the village he knew was a day's journey away, a village named Qumran where he knew the people would take them into their community, giving shelter and safety.

The morning came quickly, with Jerusalem left beyond the horizon. A weight lifted from this heart; Yosef took a deep breath of relief.

He was exhausted and so was his family. While his wife and children slept, he kept watch. They needed rest before continuing their journey. They were headed in the right direction and he knew where their destination lay.

Yosef roused his family to continue the journey. After a sleepy start, they continued on the dusty road. Yosef's exhaustion exceeded what he expected. As they moved along, the sun's rays pounded down on him, heating him from the inside out. He held Elisheva's hand and moved slowly on the road. Rivka noticed her husband's pace slowing and reached in her satchel for the small jug of water they brought with them. As she brought out the jug, Yosef collapsed.

Elisheva giggled when her father fell, her daddy could be so funny when he wanted her to laugh. Her three-year-old face broke out into laughter when Yosef hit the ground. Rivka's reaction was the opposite of her daughter's. She rushed to her husband and knelt beside him. She rolled him from his position face down onto his back. His eyes were wide and his mouth was open. She leaned over him to try to hear his breathing; no breath came from his lips. She shook him with her free hand, the other still holding Reuven. Yosef did not stir. He lay on the ground dead.

How could she continue without him? Somehow she had to.

∼

Shimon heard of the new people in the village from Yochanan, one of the Essene elders. There was a new woman and her two children that came to the community seeking refuge from the persecutions of Jerusalem by the Roman Empire.

He understood what was happening in Jerusalem was atrocious, and for the safety of this little family, he thanked God. God was the center of the community, and all things came from God to his people. Shimon was sure the woman and her children could find peace in the community as they find their way to another home.

Shimon had joined the community several years before and was now a full member of the group. He had longed to join the Essene community ever since he discovered the beliefs and practices of the group. He could not embrace the business practices of his father and the lengths the family had to go to for survival. Why couldn't everyone share their fortune for the betterment of all? This concept was foreign to his neighbors, and he had held this treasured idea in secret until he discovered his new home.

He loved his community in Qumran. He finally felt closer to God because everyone shared what they had and helped each other. Everyone had their job to do; he served the community by baking the bread; Isaac and Naomi cooked meals; Aharon made cloth. Each person in the community had a purpose and a function. No one was any more important than another. This community, he felt, was doing God's work; together they were a unit in tune, in his divine image.

Rivka, still grieving for her husband, was found and rescued by the hand of God, as she thought of Yochanan. He was a kind man; he had been out in the desert in search of a lost donkey to take back to his community. Little did he know he would come across a widow and her two small children.

When Rivka, Elisheva, and Reuven arrived in the community, they were embraced by a kindness she hadn't felt since her childhood. She didn't feel worthy to be among these people; her clothes were dirty, her face covered in mud soaked with her tears, and her children were hungry and untidy.

All of her discomfort was wiped away as she was escorted to a tent for fresh clothes, a basin of water, and food for herself and her children.

After bathing, she fell into a deep sleep. The only woman she noticed when she came into the community helped her settle and feed the children. When she awoke, Elisheva and Reuven were still sound asleep. She silently moved out of the tent and into the common area. There she saw men going about their daily chores, and some were in deep prayer. She had never known men to do such "womanly" work such as making cloth, cleaning pots, or preparing a meal. These duties were considered the work of women, and men had their own work.

Her amazement continued when one of the men approached her with a cup of water to quench her thirst. She didn't know how to accept this. Her mind reeled. What would Yosef do if he saw a strange man offer his wife water? Then she remembered, Yosef was dead. At the memory, her eyes shifted from exhaustion to the agony of grief. She gratefully accepted the cup and drank from it greedily. She didn't realize how thirsty she was. After she finished, she handed the cup back to this kind man and went back to her children.

Days turned into weeks, which turned into months. Rivka and her children were completely accepted by this community. What she initially found odd was now common. She was one of only three women in the community of one hundred. Yet women were not servile to the men; on the contrary, each had their own job for the survival of the community.

The other oddity that she had come to accept was that the women had no husbands, and no man in the group claimed either as his wife. She thought everyone had to find a mate and have children. These people believed the opposite. They lived only for God and no other.

Rivka and the women cared for the children, but some of the men also took their turns playing with each and teaching them the Word of God.

She discovered that God's Word and his will were at the center of each word, action, or thought of everyone in the community. She now knew why Yosef wanted his family to find refuge in this community: he was rescuing his family not only from the Romans, but also from the earthly traps that every human can be caught in. Yosef wanted his family to know God by living as he wants.

Rivka felt her husband's presence when she made this discovery. She was filled with joy and love for her husband and for God. Yosef didn't lead his family to this community; they were led here by God. This is where they were going to stay, to serve God, by serving the community.

A NEW PEACE

While her mother tended to her daily chores, Elisheva played with her two-year-old brother, Reuven. It was a grand day; it was her birthday. She was turning five and she wanted to shout with joy. She was proud to be her mother's helper, because Rivka was very busy these days tending to the rest of their neighbors. Every day seemed to bring something new. Elisheva was not always sure what troubled their neighbors, but each was happy after the visit with her mother.

Today was very special because Reuven was happy, and well. Two nights before Elisheva awoke to find her mother hovering over her brother. Reuven was crying so loudly, his face was as red as wet earth, but as he cried, Rivka stroked her son and whispered over him. Worried and scared that her little brother was very sick, Elisheva felt the tears roll down her cheeks. Reuven was not just her brother; he was her only friend. If something happened to him, she would be alone, as she and Reuven were the only children in the community.

As she sobbed, she closely watched her mother. She could not hear what her mother was saying, but as she stroked Reuven and spoke, his cries began to settle and slowly stopped. His breathing, which was heavy, began to lighten, and slowly a smile crept onto his chubby face. Elisheva saw the glow in his eyes from across the room, where she sat as if stuck to the floor. Her brother cooed to Rivka, who took her son in her arms and began softly singing him back to sleep.

Elisheva admired her mother so much. She had seen Rivka help make people in the community feel better, and she was grateful that she could do the same for her little brother.

She remembered that Levi, one of the younger men in the community, visited Rivka often to help teach. Levi fascinated her, he was one of the more handsome men in the village, and he was always very kind to her and Reuven. Levi taught them how to tend to a small garden. Elisheva was so proud when her garden began to grow and she could not wait to show Levi her first crop of three figs.

But today he didn't come to read the scrolls and teach. He had fallen while gathering the harvest, and as he fell a tool punctured his leg.

When he entered their dwelling, Levi's face was ashen, but his eyes had a quiet calm. Elisheva could not understand why he was so tranquil: blood gushed from his open wound! She looked quizzically at his face, so serene and peaceful.

Levi was hurt and her mother worked quickly on him. She gathered herbs and placed them on the cut. Blood drenched the floor, but Rivka quietly and expertly went about the business of healing him. Levi never flinched or complained. Elisheva had seen others complain when they were hurt, but never Levi, and this time was no different. Reuven played in the corner, completely oblivious to his mother's activity. Reuven barely noticed that Levi had entered their small home, as he was too interested in his ball made of string to be concerned with a bleeding man.

As Rivka worked, Elisheva could hear her mother's prayers over Levi's wound. She didn't know how words could help stop the bleeding, but Rivka never stopped praying as she worked on Levi's wound.

With his eyes closed, Levi's face showed deep concentration. She had seen that expression before when her brother tried to carry out something he had never done in his two-year-old life.

Rivka also had a look of profound meditation on her face. She had a look of peace and tranquility about her; it was as if she glowed as she worked with Levi. Elisheva had not seen this before, but she had never seen a man on the floor in a pool of blood either. Nevertheless, the glow about Rivka was powerful. Elisheva could feel the energy exude from her mother and onto Levi's wound. The energy was so vast that it caused Reuven to stop what he was doing and move toward his mother. Without a command, Reuven moved close to Rivka, and in harmony with her, he began to roam his tiny hands over Levi's wound.

Elisheva had never seen her brother do anything like this before; he was generally disagreeable with any sort of command or duty, but now it was as though he was uncontrollably drawn to help heal. She too felt drawn to her mother and brother's side. She didn't understand why or what she could do, but she knew they needed her.

The wound was grisly. Flesh was torn away, exposing ripe, blackened red tissue. Herbs covered the wound, and the blood that had gushed when Levi come to them now slowed and stopped. Rivka tore an old piece of cloth and tied it around

Levi's leg. Elisheva helped lift his leg, heavy with blood, herbs, and torn flesh. Rivka wrapped the cloth and tied it so the flesh connected underneath. While she went about covering the wound, she did not stop praying and neither did Reuven. Elisheva had never heard Reuven pray or use words so completely. The energy that radiated from Rivka enveloped both Reuven and Levi.

After Levi's wound was covered, Rivka continued to move over the wound. Then as suddenly as Levi entered their home, he stood, thanked Rivka, patted Elisheva and Reuven on the head, smiled, and went back to finish his work in the field.

Elisheva sat dumbfounded. She could see his leg was weak, because he limped as he walked. She watched him from the door opening and could see him pick up his tool. Yochanan, the village elder, and Shimon gave him a stool and a burlap bag to gather what they had harvested. Levi looked relieved and grateful to be back to contributing to the success of the village in any way he could.

She looked at her mother in amazement. She had seen Rivka help other people in the village, but she never saw someone bleeding so severely, then appear well in such a short time.

"Elisheva, what are you looking at?" Rivka asked as she tended to Reuven.

"Mama, I don't understand what happened. Levi was very hurt and now he's out in the field. You made him better." She continued to look out at Levi who was putting everything handed to him in his burlap bag.

Rivka washed Reuven's face and smiled at her daughter. He giggled when she kissed his cheek and scooted him out the door.

"I didn't do anything," Rivka told Elisheva in a slightly scolding tone. "You or I or Yochanan—we do not do anything alone. God does everything. He simply uses us to do his work."

"I don't understand," Elisheva was still confused. She had watched her mother heal Levi. She couldn't see God. How can God use someone if he wasn't there? This thought puzzled the five-year-old.

"You can't understand the power of God?" Rivka moved closer to her daughter.

"No—I mean, yes, I suppose. But he isn't here; how can God use you if he is not here?"

Rivka smiled broadly. She loved the quizzical nature of her little girl. Elisheva questioned and marveled at the world around her, and that joy in discovery filled Rivka with delight.

"God is everywhere, inside all of us. And he has given each of us the power to help people feel better when they are sick or hurt, to feel great joy, like the joy your father and I felt when you and Reuven were born. We receive all of this because it is God who made us. So why wouldn't he give us the power to do what needs to be done to be happy?

"Your father led us to this village to escape the Romans who destroyed our old home and killed many people. Since we arrived here, I have been learning about healing and how God gives us the power to do his work. We people are here to learn and live in his Word, and that's just what we are doing."

Elisheva understood the words her mother said, but could not grasp how God can do what she said; it didn't make sense.

Rivka saw the confused look on Elisheva's face. "Come with me and let's tend to the meal." Elisheva looked up at her mother and smiled broadly, she loved helping her mother, and she put the puzzling events of the day out of her mind.

The days passed, one into another, season after season. Rivka absorbed everything she could about the power of healing. She sat with Yochanan as often as she could so he could impart everything he knew to her. The more time she spent with Yochanan, she discovered she could not recall everything he said, so one evening after her children slept, she brought parchment and a writing tool with her so she could scribble down what Yochanan told her.

Occasionally when Yochanan and Rivka met, Shimon and Levi would join them and add their thoughts to Rivka's journal. As time passed, Rivka found she had more pieces of parchment than she could carry. When she filled a new parchment, she stored each piece in an urn that she stored in a cave for safekeeping.

The caves were cool, safe, and nearby. She enjoyed the walk to the cave and the time she spent there. She felt God was physically present when she would deliver her precious parchment to the urns in the cave. She felt she was visiting with God each time she read the parchments.

One afternoon she decided Elisheva was old enough, at seven, to go with her on her walk to deliver another parchment. Reuven was now five and went out to the fields to do his five-year-old part. He felt like he was one of the men when he would go with Levi to the field. Rivka was so proud of her son; he was growing into a fine young man, one that Yosef would be proud of. As she watched Reuven trot off to the field, she took the latest parchment, a wrap for her and Elisheva, and headed toward the caves.

Rivka held her daughter's hand as they walked. She talked about God and her work with Yochanan. Her eyes were bright with delight as she shared her knowledge with Elisheva, who absorbed every word, asking questions and repeating what was told so she could better recall it later.

When they reached the cave, Rivka placed her latest parchment with the rest.

"Mama, what are all of these urns doing here?" Elisheva asked as she scanned the cave.

"For a long time I have been talking with Yochanan and others about healing. Inside each urn are papers that I can use with the others in the community to teach them more about healing."

"But, what about . . ."

"You?" Rivka finished for her daughter. "The reason I wrote down as much as I could is so I could teach you and Reuven. You are at just the right age to begin your education."

Rivka gleamed with joy as she gazed at Elisheva, who was so happy that she would finally be able to do what her mother did for Levi that day so long ago.

There were four urns in the cave; each filled with parchments. Elisheva walked to one and took out its contents. She marveled at what she read and had to ask Rivka for help on some words as she had just learned to read.

They enjoyed their time together. Rivka placed her arm around her little girl as they read. Rivka told Elisheva what she had learned and shared healing techniques.

It was a bright day and the sun peaked into their sanctuary. Soon they would have to leave to help prepare the evening meal. At that moment, their joy was shattered by the sounds of bloodcurdling screams from the village below.

"Mama! What was that?!" Elisheva was frightened.

In a moment the mood shifted from tranquility to terror.

"Stay here!" Rivka commanded. She moved to the edge of the cave opening to witness utter horror.

Roman soldiers, horses, swords and arrows, were overrunning the village and the people she loved. Horses trampled huts, and soldiers dragged out those inside, slashing their throats and stabbing them in the chest to ensure their victims could not rise. Those who could run were chased and beaten with iron-spiked clubs.

Rivka thought she had escaped Roman brutality when she and her family fled Jerusalem. She was deadly wrong. Screams echoed up to the caves. Elisheva was whimpering in the corner, too terrified to move. She covered her ears to block out the sound of the screams and death rising from the village.

Rivka slowly backed away from the cave opening to comfort her daughter. As she moved, her eyes went wide and wild. She held back a scream as she could see her beloved son Reuven impaled by a lance, his limp body tossed aside as the soldiers continued to destroy the village and everyone in it. She could feel her heart tear apart. Her beloved son lay lifeless in the field, where he was so proud he could be of help to the men.

She wanted to rush to him, destroy his murderers and exact revenge on them and their families. Her eyes stung with anger and helplessness. It was then she heard Elisheva's sobs and knew her place was with her daughter. Rivka inched her way to comfort her child and wait until the brutes moved on away from the destruction and death they brought.

Day turned to night and another day into another night before Rivka felt it was safe to leave the cave. Only by the grace of God did the Romans pass by the caves. She wanted to protect her daughter from the devastation below, but knew they had to leave, if for no other reason than they needed more water and food. The small rations they brought with them did not last long, but Rivka wanted to be sure the Romans had left and were not coming back.

They made their way back to their little village; each carried two urns filled with parchments. Rivka directed her daughter to keep her head down and also covered Elisheva's eyes. No one should see this death, especially a little girl. All their friends were gone, so was her little boy, his life pierced by a soldier who had as much regard for Reuven's life as he would a piece of rotten meat.

As they moved through their destroyed village, Rivka picked up supplies. She took a wagon, some cloth, food and water. She took whatever she could, as they would have to journey to another place.

Rivka was inconsolable as they left their home. She looked up to God and asked for guidance and help. She fell to her knees and begged for God's grace. She clutched her daughter as she cried out. As she continued her exhausted prayer, God-given peace flowed into her body. She felt God's presence and power throughout every inch of her being. God's supremacy and love absorbed her and Elisheva, who looked up at her mother.

"Mama, God is with us, I can feel him. He has not abandoned us. You were right; God is everywhere and inside us." She smiled up at her mother and patted her hand. For a change, Elisheva comforted her mother, and Rivka let out a cry for her son, for her husband, and for her village. Her daughter's comforting words came from the mouth of God.

In Elisheva's seven years, her life had changed drastically—and it would again. She didn't know where they would go, who they would meet, but one thing stayed with her, she and her mother would continue healing anyone in need and spread the Word of God.

She also vowed to teach her children to heal, so what happened to their little village would never happen again.

Two

The Dead Sea Scrolls, the Essenes' Healing, and Spiritual Warfare

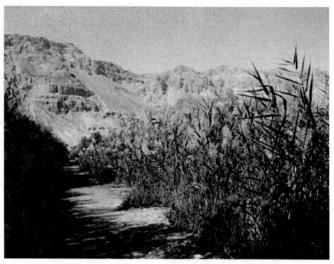

Wilderness Area at Ein Feshka Facing the Dead Sea

THE ESSENES

THE VARIOUS political upheavals during the second and first centuries bce, and then the instability that led to the Jewish revolt and the fall of Jerusalem in 70 CE had an impact on the Jews, an impact that dispersed them in many directions. One of these directions was the community of the Essenes.[1] This was the group that rescued Rivka and her children. It was a community that originated in the Jewish faith during the second century BCE. The first-century CE historian Josephus said there were 4,000 Essenes throughout the Jewish communities. The most well documented group of Essenes in Israel ate, prayed, and lived together in a monastic-type community called Qumran on the west side of the Dead Sea.

One translation for the word *Essene* is "healer." *Webster's Revised Unabridged Dictionary* (1913) understands the root as the Chaldean or Hebrew word "to heal," which corresponds with the Greek name that Philo used for the group in Egypt: *Therapeutae*. Some scholars believe the name comes from an Aramaic word that means "pious ones." Their mission was to pray for the end times and to lead holy lives to hasten the arrival of the Messiah and the true High Priest. Also central to their mission was the study the Law and healing those in need. Their apocalyptic worldview may have and perhaps did seem outrageous, but given the times of the Roman Empire and their method of conquering every ruler and territory in sight, this pious group of Jews were not far off the mark.

1. For a brief overview of the scholarly consensus on this group, see the articles "Dead Sea Scrolls" and "Qumran Community, Essenes, and Therapeutae," in Everett Ferguson, *Backgrounds of Early Christianity,* 2nd ed. (Grand Rapids, MI: Eerdmans, 1993), pp. 436–45, 487–97. The understanding of the Essenes' healing and spiritual warfare that is presented in this book comes out of the authors' own reading of various Essene writings found in the Dead Sea Scrolls.

As a monastic type of community, it was mostly men who populated the Essenes, and therefore, not many children were present. Women were allowed within the group, but marriage appears to have been forbidden as a code of their monastic lifestyle.

Our fictional heroine, Rivka, was fortunate that the Essenes did not turn away widows or children, otherwise she may have been a meal for the desert wildlife. Lovingly, the Essene community embraced all, but they did need to uphold the rules of community, and newcomers had to adopt the strict lifestyle.

The communal lifestyle of the group held that all things belonged to the community and that in loving one another, one must show kindness to all of God's creatures. But the group was always the most important. The individual played a role only as a part of the group, not as a sole entity.

All jobs in the agricultural community were held in the same esteem as any other. The leaders of the group were no more important than the baker, miller, or sweeper. In addition, the Essene people felt so committed to this way of life they rejected anything that may offend God.

Today's culture stands in sharp contrast to the Essene community. In parts of the Western world, the individual is held to be the highest, leaving the group not valued at times. An individualist society, where technological booms and inventions are so highly prized, where the individual is so praised, loses much in terms of community.

Tangible Help

For example, if a pregnant woman came to the Essenes and shared that her problem was a need for $1,500 prenatal care, the group would pool their funds together and raise what was necessary. There would be no promissory note written, no "what will you do for me?" attitude, just work for the common good—getting this woman what she needed. This attitude, and action, is what God would want, and therefore the Essene community would give in action.

In today's world, if the same woman came to her church or friends, a common response from these people may be, "we'll pray for you." Prayer is powerful and necessary for communing with God, but the Essenes took it a step further, by supporting their prayers with action. God is a God of intention *and* action. "If a brother or sister is without clothing and in need of daily food, and one of you says to them, 'God in peace, be warmed and be filled,' and yet you do not give them what is necessary for their body, what use is that? Even so faith, if it has no works, is dead, being by itself" (Brit Hadasha James 2:15–17). We must be intentional people who love and serve God! This was the model the Essene community left as a legacy to us.

Direct Dealing with Interpersonal Problems

Another contrast between the Essene community and our Western worldview can be seen in how this group managed problems. When people in the group have a problem, say, our fictional Rivka had a problem with Naomi, she would take her problem to Naomi. They would discuss the issue and resolve it. There was no passive-aggressive "we'll talk about it when I get angry enough in three years" attitude. If a resolution wasn't possible, they would bring in others. And if that didn't work, then Rivka would go to the community elders. This matches the Brit Hadasha/New Testament model:

> if your brother sins against you, go and reprove him in private; if he listens to you, you have won

your brothers. But if he does not listen to you, take one or two more with you, so that BY THE MOUTH OF TWO OR THREE WITNESSES EVERY FACT MAY BE CONFIRMED [Deut. 19:16]. And if he refuses to listen to them, tell it to the church; and if he refuses to listen even to the church, let him be to you as a Gentile and a tax-gatherer. Truly I say to you, whatever you shall bind on earth shall have been bound in heaven; and whatever you loose on earth shall have been loosed in heaven. Again I say to you, that if two of you agree on earth about anything that they may ask, it shall be done for them by My Father who is in heaven. For where two or three have gathered together in My name, there I am in their midst. (Matthew 18:15–20)

Unfortunately, although kind confrontation is extremely biblical, it is often replaced with resentment and anger—two tools the Enemy uses to put a wedge in our lives and slip in.

Problem resolution doesn't begin with "discussing" the other person, spreading the hostility; it begins by taking the grievance to the individual and sorting it out. Many readers know this, but still so few of us actually take issues to the source. Much damage is done in the name of third-person "processing."

Healing, Faith, and Prayer

Direct interaction, in contrast, leads to healing relationships, and healing was an essential part of the Essene community. People today often do not believe that healing can be a part of life (other than the healing that comes in a prescription bottle). Today, many Westerners don't trust spiritual or emotional healing. Nevertheless, all aspects of our lives are interconnected, including the spiritual. Believing prayer does have power to heal.

In addition to distrust of spiritual healing, too many in Western culture have come to think of themselves as victims. Being a victim has become chronic and a tool of Satan. So people fail to exercise faith, to pray, and to make use of all the resources for healing that are available. People believe their lives are so chaotic that they don't fit prayer into them. Rather than fitting our lives around prayer, we fit prayer around our schedule. But if we make prayer our first recourse, believing that power is available, so many lives can be transformed.

Healing as a Process

Healing is a process. The body is not magically cured by words or actions—though cures can come through miracles. Depending on the illness, modern medicine can do many "miraculous" things to help people become well. For the Essenes, however, laying on of hands was the miraculous, as they became living conduits of God's healing, literally.

Healing was a calling for the Essenes, a way of life, and anything that took away from life was considered a cause of illness. So what takes away from life? To the Essene, God is life, so the answer is the same as the answer to the question, What takes away from God? Nothing; one cannot take from an all-powerful God. But one can choose not to give—not to give trust, or belief, not to give their life choices. This worldview finally leads to the fact that perhaps illness is caused by living for one's own self and not for God.

Saying that illness can be caused by living for oneself rather than for God is not necessarily to say that God did not cause the person to be ill, for his own mysterious reasons, for he is a God of profound mysteries. Nor are we insinuating that God is punitive, punishing anyone who does not give their life totally to him. We are saying, however, that maybe the hostility and venomousness of everyday life could literally cause illness. The Essenes believed that the cure was to give these things, these grievances to God, and the process of doing so was healing. But there is a fight with the forces that try to keep this healing from happening—this is spiritual warfare. The Essenes knew this reality well. In summary, there are three reasons a person may be kept in illness:

1.   The ill person has not yet worked through the issues—either spiritual/emotional or physical—that brought on the disease.

2.   The ill person doesn't believe he or she can be healed; and/or

3.   God has a reason for the illness.

Many of these explanations and Essene virtues can be found in the Dead Sea Scrolls.

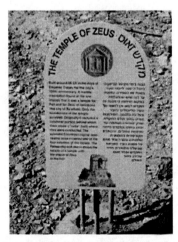

Marker for Ancient Temple of Zeus and Pan Near the Remains of the City of Banyas, Northern Israel, at the Foot of Mt. Hermon

THE DEAD SEA SCROLLS

To read the scrolls initially seems a little daunting; in reality they are not that difficult to read. We want to first discuss what they are and the amazing history behind them. Many of you already know the story; it starts with a boy . . .

It is 1947, and a small tribe of Bedouins is living on the northwest end of the Dead Sea. On one very average day for these migratory people, one of their own small children, a boy, discovered scrolls hidden within clay jars in the caves of what we now call Qumran. Over the next year, seven of these scrolls made their way from the Bedouin boy—who had no idea what he had found—into the hands of scholars. One of these scrolls was a very decent copy of the book of Isaiah; it ended up being the oldest complete manuscript of Hebrew Scripture ever found.

Also within these seven scrolls is the document first called the *Manual of Discipline,* now known as the *Community Rule,* a set of living standards for the community that lived in the area between 150 BCE and 70 CE. These dates, as well as the description of Josephus, a well-known first-century CE Jewish historian, seem to indicate that these people were the Essenes, a Jewish monastic group whose existence is documented by a range of sources. There is still some controversy over whether or not these people were the Essenes, but it is our opinion that they were.

Over 900 scrolls were found in the caves. It is important to note that every Old Testament book except the book of Esther has been found at Qumran. What this means is that this was a sound Jewish group, deeply rooted in their love for the Hebrew God and Scripture. An incredibly devoted people, one difference between them and other Jewish sects of the time, such as the Sadducees (with whom they shared in common some understandings of the Temple and the priesthood), was that the Essenes seem to be "Spirit" based. For the purposes of this book, several manuscripts from a wide range of the scrolls will be discussed to show the true connection between spiritual warfare, healing, and the sacred methods of the Essenes.

As you read the scrolls, there are several key words to understand to make the text come alive. First, the "Instructor": this word refers to the person conducting healing, a minister or teacher within the community who instructs on spiritual warfare, a sage, if you will. As you read these passages, imagine an old man with a long beard passing on wisdom from generations past, the secrets of defeating the demonic, as a group of Essenes sit by vast fires on a cold, moonlit night off the coast of the Dead Sea.

Finally, we want to discuss the credibility of the scrolls themselves. There is much, much, debate on the meaning and interpretation on much of the scrolls. We as the authors are taking a somewhat radical view on various points that other scholars might disagree with. Know that we have taken careful consideration in every theological point we make, and are sensitive to the critical nature of these writings. Nonetheless, the scrolls are important because they are the oldest record of the Hebrew Bible and other ancient texts. The Scriptures found at Qumran are probably the form of the Hebrew Bible best known to the early church. As such, they provide the basis of both Jewish and Christian belief systems; they are the basis of a spectrum of belief systems within the Judeo-Christian community.

AUTHORITY OVER THE DEMONIC IN THE FRAGMENTS

4Q510–511 Fragment 1: "Songs of the Sage for Protection Against Evil Spirits"[2] 4 And I, the Instructor, proclaim His glorious splendor so as to frighten and to ter[rify] 5 all the spirits of the destroying angels, spirits of the bastards, demons, Lilith, howlers, and [desert dwellers ...] 6 and those which fall upon men without warning to lead them astray from a spirit of understanding.

Fragments 48–49: 2 the praises of His righteousness, and ... by His mouth he frightens [all the spirits] ...

4Q560 3 [... I adjure you, all who en]ter by the body.... I adjure you by the Name of the Lord, "He who *removes iniquity and transgression*" *(Ex. 34:7), O Fever-demon and Chills-demon and Chest-pain demon* [... You are forbidden to disturb by night using dreams or by *day during sleep, O male Shrine-spirit and female Shrine-spirit, O you demons. . . ."* (italics in original)

These fragments clearly reflect the authority of the Instructor to proclaim the praises of God in relation to the demonic realm. The language is strong, reflecting an authoritative tone that gives the instructor the right to proclaim the splendor or glory of God, which the demonic entities are

2. All quotations from the Dead Sea Scrolls are from Michael O. Wise, Martin G. Abegg Jr., and Edward M. Cook, *The Dead Sea Scrolls: A New Translation,* rev. ed. (San Francisco: HarperSanFrancisco, 2005).

scared of. Thus, we have our first lesson in what scares the demonic: it is the praise of God, done with authority, no fear.

We see this same principle today in such phrases as "in the name of Jesus," evident in references from the Brit Hadasha/ New Testament (Mark 9:38–40; 16:17). There is much to be said about the fear driven into the demonic by proclaiming the glory of God. Speaking the very name of God proclaims his authority. Thus the Qumran text lines up with Brit Hadasha/ New Testament writings. This concept in the Scrolls proves that the Essenes practiced spiritual warfare from a "biblical" point of view.

MORE THAN CASTING OUT DEMONS

In looking deeper at the Gospel according to Mark, when the Legion of demons in the Gerasene demoniac trembled at Jesus' presence, he commanded that they enter the swine (Brit Hadasha Mark 5:13). What must be observed in the account is that after the Legion of demons is cast into the swine, "those who tended them ran away and reported it in the city and out in the country. And the people came to see what it was that had happened" (Mark 5:14). When the witnesses return with people from the whole surrounding area, the man who was demonized is acting quite normal. How much time was there for these people to go and gather others to see this amazing feat? Hours? Days? No, it would have taken a week, maybe two. During this time the formerly demonized man could have had a lot of healing, counseling, instruction on change of life skills, so he would not wind up with an invitation for demonic revisitation.

Just casting out a demon isn't enough. Changing behaviors, habits, thought patterns, and sometimes even belief systems is necessary to really find a place of living in God's will. Unfortunately, when the casting out of demons becomes the primary objective, it becomes a show or magic trick that is close to mockery or blasphemy.

Think of it like this: There is an angry man, therefore his state of being gives a demon of anger a legal right into his life. Now some modern teachings on spiritual warfare tell us to cast the demon out first. Fine, except what will keep anger from having a legal right to enter back in? Nothing. Here is the misconception: demons do not cause emotion, such as anger. This would impose on free will, God's greatest gift to us. As a universal law the demonic cannot touch this. But they can tamper with our emotions if we, in our free will, choose to be angry. We can give them a right to whisper lies into our ears as if it were the truth of our own minds. This is torture. So, in war, one must heal an emotion from a psychological level first, to cut off any legal right of influence the demonic might have. Then it is safe to deal with casting the demon to the Abyss.

Jesus practiced this, though it might not be apparent from Scripture until you look closer and see that he indeed also healed emotions.

THE ESSENES' SPIRITUAL WARFARE

The Essenes knew this model. There were two specific ways the Essenes practiced spiritual warfare: (1) incantation in the name of God, YHWH, and (2) prayer to God. Fragment 4Q560, quoted above, is incantation to God. It is the same model as calling on the name of Jesus in commanding the demonic to the foot of the cross. Here is an example of the second approach, an Essene prayer:

11QPs a XIX, 1–18
"Plea of Deliverance," Lines 13–16
Forgive my sin, O Lord,
and purify me from my iniquity.
Vouchsafe me a spirit of faith and knowledge,
And let me not be dishonoured in ruin.
Let not Satan rule over me,
Nor an unclean spirit;
Neither let pain nor the evil inclination
Take possession of my bones.

This prayer could be called an Essene version of the Lord's Prayer. The similarity can be seen when the two are read closely and compared. Thus, both of the Essenes' methods were used by Jesus in the Brit Hadasha/New Testament.

Pray, then, in this way:
"Our Father who art in heaven,
Hallowed be Thy name.
Thy kingdom come.
Thy will be done,
On earth as it is in heaven.
Give us this day our daily bread.
And forgive us our debts, as we also have forgiven our debtors.
And do not lead us into temptation, but deliver us from the evil one.
For Thine is the kingdom, and the power, and the glory, forever. Amen."
(Matthew 6:9–13 NASB + v. 13 footnotes)

Before we can discuss further the methods of healing used by the Essenes, we want to establish from the scrolls themselves that demons are real and present.

DEMONIC ENTITIES IN THE SCROLLS

The main function of all the demonic entities is to terrify, to lead astray, or deceive. Usually the name of the entity tells its function, as listed in the table below:

Name of Demonic Entity	Location	Action Caused
Lilith	4Q560	Terror to men
Howler	4Q560	Night terror
Chills demon	4Q510–511	Sickness
Chest pain demon	4Q510–511	Heart Attack
Male Shrine Spirit	4Q560	Idolatry
Female Shrine Spirit	4Q560	Idolatry

Three

Demons in Jewish Theology

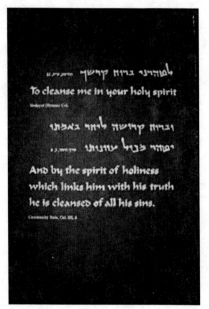

לטהרני ברוח קודשך
To cleanse me in your holy spirit

וברוח קודשה ליחר באמתו
יטהרו בכול עוונותו
And by the spirit of holiness
which links him with his truth
he is cleansed of all his sins.

Citation on Plaque at Qumran Visitors' Center

THE FOLLOWING is a brief explanation of demons, along with details about a few specific ones. We want the reader to see that these things have an ancient history, with roots in Jewish theology. Most of the descriptions below come from the Jewish tradition. Demons have been around since nearly the beginning; Jewish communities identified them and recorded how to deal with them. Yes, Jesus reportedly broke the hold of the Enemy, but they were causing pestilence before Jesus' time, and God always was and is more powerful. Thus, Jewish documents on the subject have relevance and deserve respect. It is important to be educated about the Enemy—not to know him personally, obviously—but to know his tactics. The more one understands who and what the Enemy is, the more one appreciates healing, spiritual warfare, and the tools the Essenes passed on to us.

DESCRIPTIONS OF DEMONS

There are six things said about demons found in the Talmud (a collection of ancient rabbinic writings considered authoritative for orthodox Judaism). These six things can be grouped into two categories: the similarities of demons to ministering angels, and their similarities to human beings.

Similarities to angels:

- They have wings.
- They fly from one end of the world to another.
- They can perceive the future beyond the supernatural curtain.

Similarities to human beings:

- They eat and drink as do people.
- They sexually reproduce as humans do.
- They die.

It is important to note, however, that demons are not equal to men or angels; they sit in between, with their main role being to cause harm and pestilence. Thus, Jewish sources inform us to be wary of them, as they sit in quantity among us. As they gather in great numbers, many unexplained "phenomenon" are attributed to the mischief of demons. For example, the lack of concentration coming upon a rabbi or a professor in mid-speech would be attributed to demons. Specifically, the weakness found in one's knees has long been considered to be a demon causing harm. A demon is also easily mistaken for a person under the right circumstances, deceiving individuals when it can. Discerning what is demon and what is human then becomes something to be wise about, and cautious.

THE CREATION OF DEMONS

According to one Jewish theory, God created demons but they procreated through Adam and Eve. "During the entire period of one hundred and thirty years that Adam separated himself from Eve (after the expulsion from Eden), the male spirits became impassioned through her and she bore from them; and the female spirits became impassioned through him and bore from him" (*Genesis Rabbah* 20.11). The demons and spirits procreated in this one-hundred-and-thirty-year period of separation can be grouped in two categories:

- Demons with no bodily form
- Demons called "Lilin," taking the form of human beings, but with wings

Another Mishnaic tradition says demons were created during the twilight between the sixth and seventh days of creation (*Aboth* 5.6).

MORE ON NAMES AND SPECIFIC TASKS OF DEMONS

Demons are in fact given specific names and functions. The following are examples of demons and their functions in Talmudic literature. For each one of these demons a whole book could be written, but our goal is to name the functions to help give discernment of demonic influences in your life and the lives of those around you. Later, more detail is given on what we believe are more influential demonic forces:

- **Ashmadai:** the king of demons
- **Jonathan:** one that can recite learned speeches, fooling people into thinking they are hearing godly wisdom, when it is actually mixed with demonic messages
- **Shedim:** foreign gods; the name is related to the Akkadian word *sedu*
- **Se'irim:** hairy demons also associated with foreign deities
- **Lilith:** a child-stealing demon (first wife of Adam)
- **Mavet:** related to a Canaanite underworld god
- **Rasheph:** also a Canaanite god, known in biblical literature as the god of the plague
- **Dever:** pestilence
- **Azazel:** demon thought to live in the wilderness

Demons can also perform functions such as creating lice, but they seem to have difficulty creating anything bigger.

Mixing with demons is forbidden in the Torah, even in the oldest book of laws, the Book of the Covenant; Israel is forbidden from anything pagan. But we do still see references to demons in the Talmud: In one account a demon was forced into a Roman caesar's daughter and only left when visited by the Rabbi R' Shimon; thus giving favor to the Jews under Roman authority. We also read that Abraham named the sons of his concubine after demons. Where the Talmud shares stories about the use of demons, one can conclude that they were used in accordance to God's will, in congruence with the teaching of the TaNaCH/Old Testament.

THE SHEDIM

The name of this group of demonic entities comes from a root word that can mean "to wound." They are Kabalistic in nature and known to send pestilence. Information about the Shedim shows the influences of Chaldean mythology.

Evil Deities Known as Shedu in Chaldean Culture

Chaldean writings refer to *shedu* (plural = *shedim*), a term that in this context seems to mean "Storm Demons." The Shedim are known in both Chaldean and Jewish cultures; in both the terms refer to a presence that is meant to disrupt and harm.

The "Destroyer" or Abaddon (a Shedim demon)

Abaddon means "doom" in Hebrew. In the Dead Sea Scrolls, the term refers to a place, "The Sheol of Abaddon." This demon is understood to be the King of Locusts and the Angel of the Abyss in some interpretations of Brit Hadasha Revelation 9:2–11 (see v. 11). The Acts of Thomas refers to Abaddon as a demon, or possibly the Devil himself.

This demon is believed to be the same as Asmodeus from the Book of Tobit, who slew seven husbands of Sarah, Raguel's daughter (Tobit 3:8). Carnal desire characterizes this demon. The Jews as well as the Chaldeans viewed this class of demon as one sent to be pestilent. Specifically, it is characterized by carnal desire, that is, killing husbands—not just killing anybody, but killing husbands or disrupting relationships.

This entity is referred to as the "Destroyer" in Satanism. The Destroyer is also a demon of early British paganism. During wartime, burning soldiers alive would summon its spirit.

In modern day, Abaddon is the "Destroyer," agreeing with European paganism and the live sacrifices of soldiers. This demon's responsibilities are to disrupt and kill. In the West this would be done best by attacking the family. Considering that the divorce rate in the church is fifty percent and possibly rising, it can be easily said that a destroying angel is doing the damage.

The Destroyer holds a high position, as it is known as a "King" and is the namesake of Sheol. It can be assumed that there are demons under this principality. It disrupts everything, and probably has help in the process, other Shedim. Abaddon could very well be the "Destroying Angel" and the head of all Shedim, what we believe Revelation calls locusts (Revelation 9:2–11).

A COMPARISON OF LILITH AND JEZEBEL

Lilith (First Wife of Adam)

Lilith is a very interesting topic of discussion. She, according to a Jewish tradition, was the first wife of Adam, not Eve. If you read Genesis closely, it is not said Eve is the first wife. Adam, however, disputed with Lilith for various reasons, one of them being sexual (she wanted to be on top, proving her domination over Adam). Lilith wanted control over Adam, and the domination issue split her and Adam apart. Then, even though Adam wanted her to stay in the Garden after she had run away, Lilith refused. She chose to leave the Garden of Eden by uttering the secret name of God, eventually leading to her banishment. She then mated with a demon called Samuel, making hundreds of demon offspring. Adam pleaded for her, and God sent three angels to bring her back. But she refused, mutated into something demonic herself, and was banished to the bottom of the Red Sea.

Till this day, Jews in Israel put charms with angels on them while their firstborn males sleep, to keep away Lilith, who is responsible for killing firstborn males. In summary, in every instance Lilith rebels against God and rebels against Adam.

Lilith as a Demon

Lilith is believed to harm male children and is the mother of all incubi and succubae (demon seducers). Isaiah 34:14–15 describes her as a "screech owl" or vampire. Jewish exiles in Babylon knew her as a "goddess of the night."

The "Song for a Sage," in the Dead Sea Scrolls, lists her among other demons to be prayed against, agreeing with Isaiah 34:14. Other texts found at Qumran, including "The Seductress," cite her as a "strange woman" whom they warn about, paralleling Proverbs 2 and 5. Lilith is also considered to be the lover of Satan and the "Queen of Hell."

Jezebel

It is also interesting to look at the life of Jezebel, asking whether it is possible that a demonic influence led by Lilith influenced her. Jezebel was a Phoenician queen and seductress who turned King Ahab away from Jehovah. As queen of the Northern Kingdom of Israel, she encouraged temples of Baal in Israel and slaughtered the prophets of the Lord. She controlled Ahab, subjecting Israel to tyranny.

After Ahab died, Jezebel ruled through her son Ahaziah. Then when Ahaziah died in battle, Jezebel exercised control through her son Joram. Finally, when Joram was killed by Jehu, Jehu had her servants kill Jezebel, and her corpse was eaten by dogs, fulfilling Elijah's prophecy.

Again, in every instance, we see rebellion against God and rebellion against her husband.

Comparison between Lilith and Jezebel

The actions of Jezebel parallel the actions of Lilith in two main ways: (1) rebellion against men—her husband—and (2) rebellion against God. Thus, it would appear that before there was a "spirit of Jezebel," there was a "spirit of Lilith." Besides the obvious points of rebellion against God and husband, Jezebel manipulates and harms her own sons for power. This also sounds like Lilith, considering her assignment is against male children.

The point we are trying to make is that much can be learned from the Jewish understanding of spiritual warfare, with Lilith being evidence of this.

BANISHING DEMONS IN JEWISH THEOLOGY

The question that remains is what to do when demons are present. Repeating phrases such as the following were believed to banish demons that meant to harm:

> Thou were closed up; closed up were you. Cursed, broken, and destroyed be Bar Tit, Bar Tame, Bar Tina as Shamgaz, Mezigaz, and Istamai. (*b. Shabbat* 67a)

For a demon of the privy one was to say:

> On the head of a lion and on the snout of a lioness there is the demon Bar Shirika Panda; at a garden-bed of leeks I hurled him down, [and] with the jawbone of an ass I smote him. (*b. Shabbat* 67a)

Demons were an everyday pestilence to the ancient Jew, and they were dealt with intentionally. They were believed to live in narrow and shady places, even in the toilet room. Whenever one had to go into these places, battling in spiritual warfare was an everyday occurrence. Though they seem unconventional, Jews found these methods to work long before modern-day Christians found their own methods.

THE POWER OF LOVE

There is one method that works every time in the battle against demons, evil, and the negativity of life, and that is pure love. It is the original conqueror of death in the Garden of Eden. When Eve eats from the forbidden tree, the price for disobedience—a.k.a. sin—is death. She must die according to God's own law. And for an undetermined period, possibly moments, possibly days, Adam is sinless. But Adam loves Eve. He has pure, complete love for her, and as she offers him the fruit he joins her in the sentence of death. But God in his infinite mercy sees Adam's love and so, instead of killing them, banishes them from the Garden. This is the first recording of love overcoming death.

The contrary happens when Cain kills Abel. We never really understand the problem with Cain's sacrifices, but we do understand his hatred and jealousy. This is manifested in the complete opposite of love, and death then ensues.

Ultimately, the life story of Jesus is about love overcoming death. The hold and power of evil is nothing compared to the freedom of love.

Four

Applying the Essenes' Ancient Traditions Today

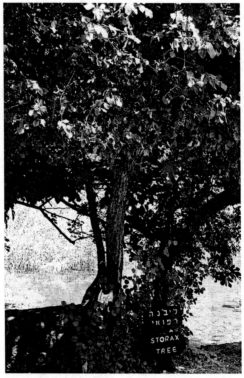

Medicinal Storax Tree, Caesarea Philipi, Israel

MODERN TEACHINGS ON SPIRITUAL WARFARE

WE HAVE established that the Dead Sea Scrolls contain teaching on spiritual warfare and we have discussed the connection between it and the methods of Jesus. We have listed the names of demons in the Dead Sea Scrolls. In addition, we presented some techniques and aspects of spiritual warfare from a Jewish standpoint. All of this has been done to give respect to and show the relevance of the Essenes; as Jews they had the background in dealing with the demonic. They took it a step further, however, and used the power of love, becoming effective tools and conduits of God.

Before we further apply what we have learned from the Essenes, let us look at some false teachings on spiritual warfare today; looking at the real thing, it should become easier to identify those who are not on task.

First, many Christians hold to an erroneous concept that once they believe in Jesus, the demonic cannot affect them; they are ensconced in a sort of spiritual "Jesus bubble." In our experience, this idea comes more from Western culture than the Bible. Every Christian people group outside a Western worldview accepts that the demonic can affect anybody. The first-century Jews, Essenes, and Christians recognized the power of the demonic. However, Western Christians consider themselves immune. To put it another way, when believers in the West see believers in the East or Middle East become susceptible to demonic attack, they automatically assume that they are not "real" believers; if they were, the demonic could not touch them. This attitude is a sort of cultural elitism. Let's put culture aside and accept the possibility that Western believers are susceptible.

The "Jesus bubble" idea of immunity to spiritual attack is not logical as Jesus himself was allowed to be tempted by

Satan. Three times the devil tried to lure Jesus away from his mission and from God's truth to satisfy his own desires (Brit Hadasha Matthew 4:1–11). If Jesus "has been tempted in all things as we are, yet without sin" (Brit Hadasha Hebrew 4:15), then surely it is safe to say that Christians may be susceptible to demonic attack.

In addition, Westerners have emotions just like anyone else, and poorly handled emotions can be a point of entry for the demonic. As in the case of Susan, whose case we will discuss in the next section, childhood trauma, emotional illness, poor choices that led to her being stuck in unhealthy relationships can all be interconnected with demonic attachment. Either outright sin or a series of poor choices (or both) can make one vulnerable to spiritual attack or oppression.

The sad thing is that many believers assume that there is nothing to overcome, as we have this invisible "shield." It is true that we have a spiritual shield, but in free will we can choose to not use it, even as believers. So we must choose wisely; this is what both Jesus and the Essenes taught. In Matthew 12:43–45 Jesus said that when an unclean spirit is cast out of a person that evil spirit may later return to the same person—who has now cleaned up his life—and reenter the person with another seven even more wicked demons.

How can that happen? It can happen if the person hasn't shut the doors and windows against the demonic. We shut the doors and windows by learning to make better choices, establishing good habits, gaining control of negative emotions, getting rid of any sin. Among the Essenes this happened because people lived in community with standards for their life together and practices of daily prayer and Scripture reading. They held each other accountable for the way they lived; spiritual and emotional healing could take place in such a community. Casting out demons isn't enough; we also need to help people make better choices and heal the whole person. So what if we linked some of the ancient methods and belief systems to some of the problems believers struggle with today?

Demonization is a much feared and often rejected state in modern times. But if Christians believe the Bible to be the Word of God, then the ideas that either demons do not exist or that demons do not wage war against Christians would be calling God a liar.

> For our struggle is not against enemies of flesh and blood, but against the rulers, against the powers, against the world forces of this darkness, against the spiritual forces of wickedness in the heavenly places. (Brit Hadasha Ephesians 6:12)

USING THE METHODS OF THE ESSENES TODAY

It has been important throughout this book for us as the authors to distinguish between views on spiritual warfare today and how the ancients perceived it. Now we want to discuss some of the methods in a bit more detail to help you, the reader, conquer some of the demons in your own life and the lives of those you love.

This book has presented spiritual warfare as a twofold method, roughly speaking: (1) incantation using the name of God, YHWH, and (2) prayer to God. The following story, or case study, is based on real people that have come to our Healing Center for help. Though spiritual warfare is a twofold method, many techniques are involved. Throughout the story, notice these techniques, as we believe this is the best way for you to learn.

A CASE STUDY

Susan came to the office a broken woman, 48 years old, married for 25 years, with a long history of depression and suicidal tendencies. As we listened to this woman's story, we could see traits of codependency and see emotional scars left by negligent parents and by a husband who displayed narcissistic tendencies, leaving Susan empty and alone.

In her past, Susan spent about twelve years in bed, literally: missing her kids' sports games, ordering pizza for dinner just too many times. The voices in her head telling her she was worthless had become a daily event now, and those voices were demonic. Her narcissistic husband further convinced her that she was even more worthless. Yes, Susan had made mistakes; there were open doors that led the Enemy straight into her life. But on the opposite side of that coin, she did not deserve the assault that the Enemy was giving her. Which leads to a question: Was it her own behavior that opened this door for the Enemy so widely? Or did the Enemy have a foothold since she was a little girl, with dysfunctional parents, and that led her to the place of desperation?

As we worked through the emotional and psychological aspects of removing codependency and moved through the depression by giving Susan some very real tools on reversing behavior connected with it, the time came to do some inner healing, some spiritual warfare.

We begin every session by praying for protection over each person present and their families and our office itself. In other words, we pray protection over every circumstance in that room. It is a way of setting the stage for the battle to come. Once it is established that God is given control from the beginning of the session, it is then time to confront the Enemy.

This is where incantation in the name of God is used. Some believers would still call this prayer, but by definition it is incantation. We drag each demon to the foot of the cross and command it to stay there for the rest of eternity, sending no reinforcements back. We order them using the name of God, and we post angelic protection between the person and all demonic forces. We then ask if there are any demons remaining that may leave the person vulnerable to another attack. If there are any that will speak, they have to surrender to God's will; if you set the stage right by inviting the presence of God before anything else, there is no issue.

Susan had many demons come out, and over the course of several months of healing emotionally, her demons had no right to stay. If we had gone for the demonic influence in her life before dealing with some of her emotional issues, specifically her past, the results might have been disastrous. But with Susan's emotions in a place of love and understanding, the demonic had no entrance to come back in, unless invited in by Susan again. Unfortunately this sometimes happens, whether it is a person's culture or dependency issues, once in a while the demonic is literally invited back in by sin.

Some people do not want to get rid of their demons. This sounds blunt, but it can be the truth. Whether it means they have to leave an abusive situation or remove something evil from their life, sometimes people prefer to hold on to their demons—even believers. It is free will.

We know this is a very brief explanation of spiritual warfare, but hopefully it is enough to whet your appetite and enough for you to draw some of your own conclusions on spiritual warfare and its roots. It is an ancient practice, as you can see from the various Jewish sources, and its techniques are many. But what is constant is the power of love, the presence of God, and the authority of his Name. We believe he is the

Hebrew God, the God of the Jews, and Jews have been dealing with this pestilence longer than any televangelist. So take a deep look at these people, the Essenes, and how they lived and how they fought the Enemy.

The next section is about an experience we had with a house in Sedona, Arizona, a beautiful, but trippy place for those of you who have not been to it. It is a side note on spiritual protection and authority, something good to know so you do not run into the same kind of trouble we did.

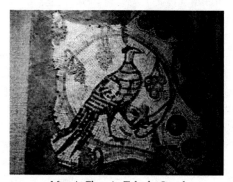

Mosaic Floor in Tabgda, Israel

SEDONA, ARIZONA

Kathleen and I (Luke) were invited to go to Sedona to help a church dealing with some demonic presences in their congregation. That was easy, as it turned out, but the house we ended up staying at almost killed us.

As we were invited to help this church deal with some of its demon issues (for lack of a better word) we ended up staying at one of the attendee's summer homes in a more remote part of Sedona. It was free, and although Kathleen and I had a bad feeling about this house even before we got there, it was still free, and we enjoy a good challenge. So off we went.

As we pulled up to the house, both of our spiritual warning signs came up. It's hard to explain, we just knew this was going to be bad news. But like I said, we enjoy a good challenge, and dealing demonic houses and their inhabitants is a favorite thing to do for us. Unfortunately we were a little prideful about it at the time, so we stayed . . .

We walked into the house with the owner, and he started explaining to us that there were no locks on the door, no phones, no Internet, no TV, and not even any hot water. But he seemed nice enough, and spiritually speaking the guy had no demons attached. We know because Kathleen has the gift of seeing into the spiritual realms (angels, demons, etc.). I (Luke) have other gifts that informed me the guy was clean, but the house was pretty much evil.

As we went to bed the first night it was relatively calm, the house was spiritually charged, but it stayed neutral anyway. Nothing tried to harm us on any level, but it was definitely an interesting night. The next day came and went with nothing unusual, but neither of us wanted to really go back to the house that night. Oddly enough, though, the second night was completely calm; we slept great. We went through the next day totally relaxed and almost excited to come back to what was pretty much just a remote cottage. Then came the third night . . .

That day was also calm, almost boring even, like we were trying to be lulled into believing we were safe. Then the time came to go "home," as we called it by then, and we started the drive back. As we entered this more remote part of Sedona, Kathleen and I felt this incredible evil just rise over us. As we pulled into the wooded area that surrounded the house things just got eerie: It was foggy all around the house, with a light mist. There was no moon that night; it was pitch black, not to mention the sheer presence of evil that we felt we were walking straight into. Then something happened I will never forget. My mind switched over to a dream that I had the previous year, where I was in a forest just like this one; you might call it déjà vu, except it was a stronger pull than even that.

In my dream I was traveling through the woods with Kathleen in a car, a black SUV. As we drove around in this black SUV (in my dream) you could see the faint lights of a house through the trees of the forest. Then all of a sudden, the SUV, in my dream, turned, and as it turned, through the lights came a form of a woman, a woman with long hair in a black dress, that was floating through the forest with a knife in her hands trying to kill us. Then I woke up!

Now I am back in the forest with Kathleen and I realize, *I am living my dream.* Everything was the same; every little detail in my dream was the reality of my circumstances. Kathleen, knowing I was having some kind of experience, looked at me and said, "we're going to die aren't we?" I answered, "I think we just might." I pulled a U-turn and we ended up staying at a five-star resort that night; she insisted that if we were going to die it was going to be in style!

Unfortunately you cannot run from the Enemy like that. We woke up the next morning and knew we had to go back and deal with whatever was in that forest. As we drove back in the morning and pulled into the forest, the evil was there waiting in the house, and we both knew it. Besides, we had to go back and get our belongings—Satan was not going to win. We reluctantly parked the car, and as we walked into the house we really had no idea what to expect. What happened next was rather shocking.

Books were flying off shelves; doors were opening and closing on their own. It was insane, and we could not do much about it. You see, the house was free, we paid nothing for it, which was the first mistake. We had no right to the house—this is a big deal spiritually. We could not clean the house, legally speaking, from a spiritual standpoint; we could only claim personal protection for ourselves and not be intimidated. But it became complicated: while I was downstairs I heard Kathleen, who was upstairs, tell me she hated me, and she heard me tell her the same. Neither of us said those words, but something else had. It even came to the point where knives were showing up on countertops sporadically, and Kathleen was convinced that I was a stranger in the house who was going to try and kill her. It was all very amusing, but eventually we got our stuff and got out of that house.

Later we found out that about one hundred yards away from the house there is Satanist worship, and further down the road lives a black witch who runs the whole thing. So here is how to avoid times like these:

Pay for the place you are using: It will give you the right to cleanse the house, hotel room, office, etc. that you're going into.

Know the area you're working and living in: There are territorial demons that love to cause evil to happen where there is an open door. The forest of our story provides a riveting example of the demonic affecting a location and the trouble we could have foreseen if we had investigated the area.

EVEN THE PLANTS OF THE FIELD

In all our counseling, prayer work, and direction, after working with thousands of people, we find that healing is very multidimensional. Not only is there the purely demonic as we saw in the house in Sedona, Arizona, there is also the psychological and emotional mixed with the demonic, as we saw in the case of Susan. In addition, the story of Rivka's healing Levi's awful gash depicts the overlapping of the spiritual with physical healing.

Rivka's healing arts, gifts, and skills were passed on to Elisheva and on down from generation to generation. Though sometimes hidden for decades due to persecution and misunderstanding, the spark lived on, and we can benefit from the knowledge of ancient healers. Nevertheless, to look at the ways of ancient people and not embrace the physical as well as the spiritual, emotional, and social would be incomplete.

Remarks by the historian Josephus reflect prevailing beliefs in the first century that illness is caused by demons, and cured through magic remedies, spells, rituals, and exorcism. Yet their cures often used plants.

Most of the plants in the Bible are native to Egypt and to what is now Israel. Some were used for ritualistic purposes, some for cooking, some for cosmetic, and many for medicinal purposes. The Old and New Testaments mention more than 125 different plants, and hundreds of them are found in many of the other Hebrew texts, the Mishnah, the Talmud, and the Midrashim.

The ancient people had to rely on the plants and herbs that they had for healing. They took what they had and used them for medicines, and to fill their gardens so that they would have them on hand in times of need. Many gardens today resemble gardens of biblical times. Most herbs—or all herbs—could be biblical, because we are told that they are for our health.

About 180 BCE the Talmud, written during this time, identified some seventy herbs and other plants as having medicinal properties—some for prevention and some for cures. This list includes everything from garlic, pomegranates, olives, dates, humen, hyssops, and many plants mainly used for food.

There were remedies for everything from high blood pressure, eye problems, hemorrhages, and intestinal ailments.

In the book of Jubilees, written in the first century BCE, we are told that the angels revealed many remedies to Noah, who recorded them in a book. A lot of symbolism is associated with various biblical plants also.

When we look at the Song of Solomon, it contains references to twenty-three plants and their products. Most of those mentioned, such as the sages, myrrh, palms, grapes, aloes, saffron, and lilies, were used for healing. Also, Jotham's parable of the trees, told in Judges 9:7–15, demonstrates the value of the fruit of the olive and fig trees and the grapevines.

A significant reference on biblical plants is Deuteronomy 8:8, which shows that the land of Israel could nourish the people with seven life-sustaining plants. It was the land of wheat and barley, of vines and fig trees, of pomegranates; a land of olive trees and honey. One thing to note here is that the honey referred to probably would not have been bees' honey, but rather the "honey" made from the nectar of the date palm tree, which is still served and sold in Israel today.

A HOLISTIC VIEW

The point is that healthy living is holistic: it is spiritual, emotional, physical. It is dynamic. And God gives us the information we need to be healthy—even down to the seeds of the earth. The Essenes knew this holistic view of health; it was spiritual science to them, and this is what we try to do today.

Our Healing Center focuses on biblical healing, striving to help individuals find wholeness and shalom in all areas of their lives. One of the cornerstones for this is the model used during the Second Temple Period in the Judean wilderness, as recorded by the Essene community in the Dead Sea Scrolls.

About the Authors

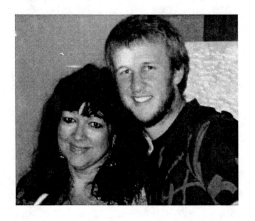

Kathleen Arai lives in Pasadena, California
Luke Rideout also lives in Pasadena, California

They can be reached through:

The Healing Center
127 No. Madison Ave, Suite 214
Pasadena, CA 91101
Telephone: 626-744-0632
Email: Healing@DeliveredSoul.com
Web: www.DeliveredSoul.com